REACTIVE ARTHRITIS DIET COOKBOOK

Healing Recipes and Nutritional Strategies for Managing Pain, Enhancing Mobility, and Restoring Wellness

IRIS JADE

© [2024] [IRIS JADE]

Reserved rights apply. Without the publisher's prior written consent, no portion of this publication may be copied, distributed, or transmitted in any way, including by photocopying, recording, or other mechanical or electronic means, with the exception of brief quotations used in critical reviews and other noncommercial uses allowed by copyright law.

DISCLAIMER

The data in the book " REACTIVE ARTHRITIS DIET COOK BOOK" is solely meant to be used for general educational purposes. Since the author is not a medical expert, none of the information in this book should be interpreted as medical advice. It is recommended that readers get individualized counsel and guidance from certified healthcare specialists regarding their particular health issues. This book's author has done every effort to guarantee that the material is accurate. However, no warranty is provided on the completeness, correctness, reliability, or applicability of the information due to the dynamic nature of medical research and the variety of individual health problems. Any mention or reference to any person, thing, website, association, or other names in this book does not imply the author's support. The author stresses that any reference of these organizations is only for informational purposes and disclaims any affiliation or association with them.

It is recommended that readers independently check and assess the information contained in this book and consult a professional when needed. Any repercussions resulting from the use or interpretation of the material in this book will not be held against the author. The reader accepts the conditions of this disclaimer by reading this book. The material of this book may be updated, changed, or revised at any time by the author to take into account new data, scientific discoveries, or advancements in medical knowledge.

Table of Contents

SECTION ONE 11

   OVERVIEW 11

   Comprehending Allergic Arthritis 11

   Dietary Interventions for Reactive Arthritis 13

   Objectives & Methodology of the Cookbook 15

SECTION TWO 19

   THE FUNDAMENTALS OF ALLERGIC ARTHRITIS 19

   Reactive arthritis: What is it? 19

   Reasons and Danger Elements 20

   Signs and Prognosis 21

   Diet and Lifestyle Importance 22

SECTION THREE 25

   MAKING A REACTIVE KITCHEN THAT IS FRIENDLY TO ARTHRITIS 25

   Putting Supplies in Your Pantry 25

Essential Utensils for the Kitchen 28

Tips for Meal Planning to Control Symptoms 30

SECTION FOUR 35

    MEDICINAL GRADE COMPONENTS 35

    Highlights of Foods That Reduce Inflammation .. 35

    The Golden Spice is Turmeric 37

    Oregano and Rosemary: More Than Just Taste Enhancers 38

    Plant-Based Omegas Found in Flaxseed and Chia Seeds 39

SECTION FIVE 41

    CREATING BALANCED MEALS 41

    Making Plates High in Nutrients 41

    Moderation and Portion Control 43

    The Value of Consistent Eating Habits 45

SECTION SIX 49

    RECIPES FOR BRUNCH AND BREAKFAST .49

Boosting Smoothies for the Morning 49

Recipes: 50

Breakfast Bowls and Parfaits Packed with Nutrition 51

Innovative and Tasty Brunch Selections 53

SECTION SEVEN 57

LUNCHES IN SUPPORT OF JOINT HEALTH 57

Bright Greens with reduced dressings 57

Healthy Stems and Soups 58

Ideas for Handheld Lunches on Busy Days 60

Personalized Trail Mix for Instant Energy 61

SECTION EIGHT 63

DINNERS THAT PROVIDE CALM 63

Filling One-Pot Dinners to Reduce Reactive Arthritis 63

Plant-Based and Vegetarian Dinner Ideas for Joint Health 65

Succulent Grilled and Roasted Treats for Cozy Dinners 67

SECTION NINE 69

SNACKS FOR COLLABORATION 69

Ideas for Nutrient-Dense Snacks to Support Each Other..69

Handmade Energy Bites and Trail Mixes 70

Including Fresh Vegetables and Fruits.................72

SECTION TEN 75

SWEETS WITH A WELLNESS ORIENTATION 75

Sugary Goodies without the Resentment 75

Luxurious yet Anti-Inflammatory Choices 79

SECTION ELEVEN 83

DRINKS TO PROMOTE JOINT HEALTH 83

The Effects of Hydration on Joint Health 83

Teas & Infusions for Healing 85

Smoothies to Refresh and Support Joints..............87

SECTION TWELVE 91

GOING BEYOND THE RECIPE BOOK 91

Including Long-Term Lifestyle Adjustments.......91

Keeping Yourself Inspired During Your Reactive Arthritis Path 94

Extra Sources and Additional Reading 96

SECTION ONE

OVERVIEW

Comprehending Allergic Arthritis

An infection in another area of the body, usually the gastrointestinal or genitourinary system, can cause reactive arthritis, a kind of inflammatory arthritis. This disorder can affect several joints, including the knees, ankles, and feet, and it frequently presents as joint pain, swelling, and stiffness. Reactive arthritis is caused by the immune system incorrectly targeting healthy joints in response to an infection; hence, understanding the underlying causes of this condition is essential for effective care. The complexities of reactive arthritis will be examined in this part, along with its causes, symptoms, and potential effects on day-to-day functioning.

Certain bacterial infections, such as those brought on by Yersinia, Salmonella, Shigella, or Chlamydia, are frequently linked to reactive arthritis. Reactive arthritis symptoms are often caused by an inflammatory response in the joints, which is initiated by the body's immune system in response to these diseases. Understanding the link between infections and inflammation of the joints is important because it informs both the treatment strategy and lifestyle modifications that can help effectively manage the illness.

Readers will have a thorough understanding of reactive arthritis after reading about the condition's symptoms and possible side effects. The wide range of symptoms emphasizes the systemic aspect of reactive arthritis, ranging from joint pain and swelling to problems like skin rashes and inflammation of the eyes (uveitis). Early diagnosis is essential for prompt action and can have a major effect on the prognosis of those who suffer from this illness.

Dietary Interventions for Reactive Arthritis

Food is an important factor in the management of reactive arthritis since some meals can either increase inflammation or improve joint health in general. In addition to medical therapies, a well-planned and balanced diet can help people with reactive arthritis live more comfortably and actively. The relationship between food and inflammation will be discussed in this section, with an emphasis on particular nutrients and dietary practices that may help reactive arthritis progress.

One factor that unites all types of arthritis, including reactive arthritis, is inflammation. To create a diet that promotes joint health, it is essential to comprehend how specific foods affect inflammation.

Whole grains, vibrant fruits and vegetables, fatty fish high in omega-3 fatty acids, and other anti-inflammatory diets can all play a significant role in reducing inflammation. Examining the scientific rationale for these dietary selections will enable readers to make knowledgeable decisions regarding their nutritional intake.

Furthermore, it is imperative to address the function of particular nutrients, including vitamin D and antioxidants, in the treatment of reactive arthritis. Vitamin D is essential for strong bones and a healthy immune system, while antioxidants can counteract free radicals, which cause inflammation. Reactive arthritis sufferers can benefit greatly from comprehensive support when these nutrients are incorporated into a well-rounded diet. In addition, discussing typical dietary errors and possible triggers will help readers make decisions that are both sustainable and beneficial.

Objectives & Methodology of the Cookbook

With its useful and delectable recipes, the "Reactive Arthritis Diet Cookbook" seeks to empower people by promoting joint health and general well-being. This section will list the cookbook's main objectives and the strategy used to accomplish them, stressing the significance of preparing meals that are both healthy for reactive arthritis management and pleasurable for daily consumption.

Objective 1: Reducing Inflammation with Nutrient-Rich Recipes

The primary objective of the cookbook is to offer a selection of dishes that emphasize lowering inflammation. Incorporating anti-inflammatory components like turmeric, ginger, and leafy greens into the meals is an attempt to improve joint health and reduce reactive arthritis symptoms. Every recipe is thoughtfully developed to achieve a balance between flavor and nutritional content, making sure that people can savor their food while enhancing general well-being.

Objective 2: Diverseness and Availability

Keeping your diet interesting and healthful requires variety. To combat this, the cookbook provides a wide variety of dishes that may be modified to suit different nutritional needs and preferences. Regardless of whether someone is on a vegetarian, vegan, or gluten-free diet, the cookbook offers solutions to suit various dietary requirements. This openness guarantees that everyone may discover tasty and nourishing meals that suit their interests, irrespective of their dietary choices.

Objective 3: Knowledge and Self-reliance

In addition to providing recipes, the cookbook educates readers about the significance of nutrition in the treatment of reactive arthritis. Every recipe includes information about the nutritional advantages of important components, enabling people to make well-informed dietary decisions. By promoting a more profound comprehension of the relationship between nutrition and well-being, the cookbook enables people to actively participate in the management of their health condition.

To sum up, the "Reactive Arthritis Diet Cookbook" offers a thorough guide to comprehending, treating, and living with reactive arthritis rather than just a compilation of recipes. Through an examination of the subtleties of the ailment, the part nutrition plays in managing it, and the objectives and methodology of the cookbook, users will set out on a path to better joint health and general well-being.

SECTION TWO

THE FUNDAMENTALS OF ALLERGIC ARTHRITIS

Reactive arthritis: What is it?

Reiter's syndrome, another name for reactive arthritis, is a form of inflammatory arthritis that arises from an infection in another area of the body, usually the genitourinary or gastrointestinal tracts. This condition typically affects the knees, ankles, and feet and is characterized by joint discomfort, edema, and inflammation. It is critical to understand that reactive arthritis is the body's immune system's reaction to an infection rather than a communicable illness. This disorder frequently affects young adults and can develop suddenly following a bacterial infection, such as a gastrointestinal or STD.

People with the HLA-B27 gene are more prone to reactive arthritis, which is frequently linked to particular genetic variables. Reactive arthritis is characterized by painful and incapacitating joint symptoms that are believed to be caused by the immune system's misdirected reaction to the infection, which in turn causes inflammation in the joints. For reactive arthritis to be effectively managed and treated, it is essential to comprehend its nature.

Reasons and Danger Elements

The main cause of reactive arthritis is infection, most frequently caused by bacteria such as Yersinia, Salmonella, Chlamydia, or Shigella. The gastrointestinal or urinary systems are usually affected by these illnesses. Reactive arthritis can result from the bacteria causing these infections getting into the bloodstream and inducing an aberrant immune response in those who are vulnerable.

Reactive arthritis develops as a result of multiple risk factors. Susceptibility is increased by genetic predisposition, namely the existence of the HLA-B27 gene. Furthermore, the chance of getting reactive arthritis may be increased by a history of specific infections, such as foodborne illnesses or STDs. It is noteworthy that not all individuals who contract these infections go on to develop reactive arthritis, and research is still ongoing to determine the precise causes of this variance in response.

Signs and Prognosis

Early diagnosis and successful treatment of reactive arthritis depend on the ability to recognize its signs. The classic symptoms, which frequently affect the lower limbs, particularly the knees and ankles, include joint pain, stiffness, and edema. Conjunctivitis, an inflammation of the eyes, skin rashes, and gastrointestinal or urinary problems are possible additional symptoms.

A comprehensive medical history, physical examination, and laboratory testing are necessary for the diagnosis of reactive arthritis. Specific antibodies can assist confirm the presence of an underlying infection, and blood tests may reveal indicators of inflammation. Imaging tests, such as MRIs or X-rays, can be used to evaluate joint damage and rule out other medical issues.

People who are suffering from the symptoms of reactive arthritis should get help as soon as possible. Timely action and improved outcomes in the management of the illness are made possible by early diagnosis.

Diet and Lifestyle Importance

Diet and lifestyle choices are crucial for controlling reactive arthritis and enhancing general health. Maintaining a healthy lifestyle helps reduce symptoms and increase the efficiency of prescribed medications. Regular exercise that is customized to each person's abilities and preferences might help to loosen up joints and lessen stiffness.

When it comes to nutrition, some foods have the potential to make inflammation worse while others may have the opposite effect. Omega-3 fatty acids, which are present in flaxseeds and fatty fish like salmon, are well-known for their anti-inflammatory properties and may help people with reactive arthritis. Berries and leafy greens are two examples of foods high in antioxidants that might help lower inflammation.

Furthermore, it's critical to maintain a healthy weight because being overweight can aggravate symptoms and put strain on joints. It is recommended to collaborate with medical specialists, such as nutritionists and rheumatologists, to create a customized food and lifestyle plan that meets each person's needs.

In summary, understanding reactive arthritis, determining its origins and risk factors, identifying symptoms for an early diagnosis, and adopting a lifestyle and diet that support general well-being are all important components of a holistic approach to managing the condition. Reactive arthritis sufferers can improve their quality of life and effectively control their inflammatory condition by taking care of these factors in a thorough manner.

SECTION THREE

MAKING A REACTIVE KITCHEN THAT IS FRIENDLY TO ARTHRITIS

Putting Supplies in Your Pantry

Overview

The cornerstone of a responsive kitchen that is arthritis-friendly is a well-stocked pantry. Making sure that your cupboard is stocked with healthful, anti-inflammatory foods can make a big difference in helping you manage your symptoms and maintain your general well-being. This is a thorough approach to filling your cupboard with goods that support a diet for reactive arthritis.

Complete Grains

Choose whole grains like oats, brown rice, and quinoa. These grains provide a steady supply of energy without inducing inflammation because they are high in fiber and other minerals. Include these grains in your diet to help maintain stable blood sugar levels and support joint health.

Pulses and Legumes

Chickpeas, lentils, and beans are great plant-based sources of fiber and protein. They can be added to soups, stews, and salads, and they make a flexible base for a variety of recipes. Legumes are important mainstays in a reactive arthritis-friendly pantry because they promote fullness and reduce inflammation.

Good Fats

Opt for oils that reduce inflammation, such as flaxseed, avocado, and olive oils. Monounsaturated and polyunsaturated fats found in these oils contribute to heart health and reduce inflammation.

To maintain their nutritious value, add them to salad dressings or cook them at a low temperature.

Spices and Herbs

Use a range of herbs and spices that are well-known for their anti-inflammatory qualities to improve the flavor of your food. Herbs like turmeric, ginger, garlic, and cilantro can enhance the flavor of your food and possibly alleviate the symptoms of arthritis. Try out different combinations to make tasty, health-conscious meals.

Goods in Cans

Stock up on canned items, such as fish packed in water, beans, and tomatoes. You can quickly and healthily create meals with these convenient and long-lasting ingredients. Verify the labels to be sure there aren't many additives or preservatives in canned products.

Gluten-Free Selections

Think about using gluten-free substitutes, such as almond flour, coconut flour, and gluten-free pasta, for people who are sensitive to gluten. These solutions minimize the chance of aggravating arthritic symptoms while meeting specific dietary needs and guaranteeing a varied and fulfilling range of meals.

Essential Utensils for the Kitchen

Ergonomic Cutlery

Invest in ergonomically designed utensils to reduce joint strain. To make meal preparation easier to access and less stressful on your hands, look for kitchen instruments with comfortable grips and handles. Using adapted kitchenware can greatly enhance your cooking experience.

Non-Slip Flooring

Put non-slip mats in high-traffic areas of your kitchen to prevent people from tripping and falling. For people with reactive arthritis, it's critical to provide a stable and safe environment. Non-slip mats add a layer of safety, particularly in the area around the stove and sink.

Cooking Appliance

In a kitchen designed for someone with reactive arthritis, a food processor can be a game-changer. It relieves the pressure on your joints by doing away with the necessity for constant chopping and slicing. Use the food processor to easily prepare fruits, nuts, and vegetables, among other things.

Cooker on the Slow Side

When energy levels are low, a slow cooker is a great complement. You can have a tasty, nourishing dinner by evening without having to give it constant care if you just toss the ingredients into the pot in the morning. This gadget cuts down on hands-on time in the kitchen and streamlines cooking.

Jar Opener

Jar opening can be difficult for people who have arthritis. To make this procedure easier, use a good jar opener. Seek for versions with movable handles that can hold different-sized jars so you can easily reach necessities in your pantry.

Tips for Meal Planning to Control Symptoms

Well-Composed and Vibrant Meals

Make an effort to prepare meals that are colorful, and well-balanced, and include a range of fruits, vegetables, lean meats, and whole grains. Strive for a plate that is as colorful as a rainbow because various tones frequently signify different nutrients that are beneficial to general health.

Oftentimes, little meals

Consider eating smaller, more frequent meals throughout the day as an alternative to heavy ones. This method can assist in controlling energy levels and avoiding weariness, which is a common problem for people with reactive arthritis. Arrange wholesome snacks to ensure a consistent nutrient intake.

Drink plenty of water.

It's essential to stay hydrated for joint health and general well-being. Incorporate hydrating meals, herbal teas, and lots of water into your meal plan. Drinks with added sugar and caffeine should be avoided since they might worsen dehydration and inflammation.

Conscientious Consumption

Savor every meal and pay attention to your body's cues when you eat mindfully. Meals shouldn't be rushed through because this can result in overheating and discomfort. Being mindful of your body during meals allows you to better understand how it reacts to various foods and recognize possible triggers.

Work Alongside a Nutritionist

Seeking advice from a nutritionist or dietitian can offer tailored recommendations for controlling reactive arthritis with food. They can assist in developing a meal plan that is customized for your requirements, taking into account your dietary requirements, preferences, and symptom management objectives.

Getting Ready in Advance

Make meal preparation easier by organizing and cooking some of your meals ahead of time. To speed up the cooking process, chop veggies, marinade proteins, and portion ingredients. This method cuts down on the amount of time and work needed in the kitchen regularly.

To sum up, designing a reactive arthritis-friendly kitchen requires making deliberate decisions about what to put in your pantry, what important cooking utensils to have, and how to organize your meals. Through the integration of these components into your diet, you can improve your general health and effectively treat symptoms.

SECTION FOUR

MEDICINAL GRADE COMPONENTS

Highlights of Foods That Reduce Inflammation

When it comes to controlling reactive arthritis with food, a key consideration is adding foods that reduce inflammation. These nutrient-dense superfoods are essential for reducing discomfort and enhancing joint health.

Selecting the Correct Vegetables and Fruits

A diet high in fruits and vegetables is considered anti-inflammatory. Packed full of vitamins, minerals, and antioxidants, they can effectively target the root cause of inflammation. Strawberries and blueberries, in particular, are prized for having high concentrations of anthocyanins, which have strong anti-inflammatory effects. Rich in vitamins and minerals, leafy greens like kale and spinach have a general anti-inflammatory effect.

Complete Grains as a Basis

An anti-inflammatory diet's main components are whole grains including quinoa, brown rice, and oats. Tightly packed with fiber, they help to regulate inflammation in addition to supporting digestive health. Whole grains provide complex carbs that release energy gradually, avoiding blood sugar spikes that may cause inflammatory reactions.

Slim Proteins for Healthy Joints

Lean protein sources such as chicken, fish, and legumes are essential for those with reactive arthritis. Red meats contain saturated fats, whereas these proteins do not. Instead, they provide vital amino acids. Particularly fatty fish, such as mackerel and salmon, provide omega-3 fatty acids, which are well known for their anti-inflammatory properties.

Spices & Herbs with Restorative Potential

For millennia, people have valued herbs and spices for their culinary uses as well as their powerful medicinal qualities. Because of their potent anti-inflammatory properties, some herbs and spices are highlighted in the context of a reactive arthritis diet.

The Golden Spice is Turmeric

Turmeric is a potent anti-inflammatory due to its key ingredient, curcumin. Turmeric, which has a characteristic golden color, is used in traditional medicine to treat joint discomfort and inflammation. Adding turmeric to food or using pills can be a tasty way to control inflammatory arthritis.

Ginger: A Quick Solace

Gingerol is a bioactive molecule with anti-inflammatory and antioxidant properties that is found in ginger, a spice known for its fiery flavor. Ginger can help reduce inflammation and potentially ease the symptoms of reactive arthritis, whether it is added to drinks or cooked as a spice.

Oregano and Rosemary: More Than Just Taste Enhancers

Herbs like oregano and rosemary not only improve food flavor but also have anti-inflammatory qualities. Compounds in these herbs may help lower oxidative stress and inflammation. Add them to marinades, sauces, or spices to enhance the taste and possibly even provide health advantages to your food.

Addition of Omega-3 Fatty Acids

Being heralded as superheroes in the battle against inflammation, omega-3 fatty acids are an essential part of a diet for reactive arthritis.

Fatty Fish to Promote Cooperation

Salmon, trout, and sardines are examples of fatty fish that are excellent providers of omega-3 fatty acids.

Due to their ability to prevent the synthesis of inflammatory molecules, these essential fats are crucial in the reduction of inflammation. Frequent ingestion of fatty fish has been shown to improve joint health and maybe reduce reactive arthritis symptoms.

Plant-Based Omegas Found in Flaxseed and Chia Seeds

Flaxseeds and chia seeds are great options for anyone who would rather obtain their omega-3s from plant sources. These seeds, which are high in alpha-linolenic acid (ALA), offer a satisfying vegetarian substitute for fatty fish. Adding chia seeds to salads or ground flaxseeds to smoothies are two easy and delicious ways to include these anti-inflammatory superfoods in your diet.

Walnuts: A Crunchy Omega-3 Source

Walnuts provide an additional plant-based supply of omega-3 fatty acids due to their unique flavor and texture. These nuts are a great way to add alpha-linolenic acid (ALA) to a variety of cuisines or just have them as a snack. A tasty way to support joint health and lower inflammation is by including walnuts in your diet.

In conclusion, anti-inflammatory foods, herbs, and omega-3 fatty acids can all be powerful allies in controlling symptoms and enhancing joint health when included in a well-designed reactive arthritis diet. Through the adoption of a wide variety of nutrient-dense foods, people can take proactive measures to reduce inflammation and improve their overall health.

SECTION FIVE

CREATING BALANCED MEALS

Making Plates High in Nutrients

A key component of the Reactive Arthritis Diet is creating nutrient-rich plates, which guarantees that people with this condition get the vitamins and minerals they need to support their general health and effectively manage their symptoms. It's critical to prioritize a variety of nutrient-dense foods that support joint health and lower inflammation while organizing meals. Every meal should include a range of vibrant fruits and vegetables, complete grains, lean meats, and healthy fats.

Including Anti-Inflammatory Foods: Including foods with anti-inflammatory qualities is one of the main objectives when creating nutrient-rich plates for reactive arthritis. Flaxseeds, walnuts, and fatty fish like salmon are good sources of omega-3 fatty acids, which can help lower inflammation. Broccoli, berries, and leafy greens are examples of colorful vegetables that are high in antioxidants, which are essential for reducing inflammatory processes.

Macronutrient Balancing: A proper proportion of carbs, proteins, and lipids characterizes a well-balanced dish. Lean proteins like chicken, tofu, or lentils promote muscle health, while complex carbs like quinoa or brown rice offer long-lasting energy. Good fats that come from almonds, avocados, and olive oil help to lubricate joints and promote general health.

Vitamin and Mineral Prioritization: People with reactive arthritis must make sure they get enough vitamins and minerals in their diet. Calcium-rich foods like kale and almonds are essential for keeping strong bones and joints, while vitamin D, which can be acquired from sources like fatty fish and fortified dairy, improves bone health. Including a range of vibrant veggies guarantees a spectrum of vital vitamins and minerals that help the immune system as a whole.

Moderation and Portion Control

Maintaining a healthy weight and controlling reactive arthritis symptoms are greatly aided by portion management and moderation. Large serving sizes might result in an excessive consumption of calories, which may exacerbate pain and inflammation. People can achieve a balance between enjoying their meals and promoting their general well-being by implementing mindful eating habits.

Techniques for Mindful Eating: Being aware of one's hunger and fullness cues is crucial for mindful eating, especially for people with reactive arthritis. Overeating can be avoided and a better relationship with food can be fostered by eating deliberately, enjoying every meal, and paying attention to your body's cues. Nutrient infusions can be sustained throughout the day with smaller, more balanced servings that don't raise blood pressure.

Tailoring Quantities to Individual Needs: Dietary needs vary greatly among people, thus it's important to tailor quantities according to individual needs. The ideal portion sizes for a certain diet or set of medical conditions can be ascertained by speaking with a qualified dietitian or healthcare provider. Moreover, maintaining a meal record could help spot trends and modify portion sizes as needed depending on how each person reacts to certain foods.

Energy Intake and Expenditure: Keeping a healthy balance between energy intake and expenditure is crucial for managing weight and general health. Frequent physical activity promotes weight regulation in addition to joint health. People can give their bodies the energy they need for daily activities without placing unnecessary strain on their joints by knowing their calorie demands and choosing educated meal choices.

The Value of Consistent Eating Habits

A key component of the Reactive Arthritis Diet is creating and maintaining regular eating patterns, which help to stabilize blood sugar levels and reduce inflammation. An irregular diet, which includes missing meals or eating a lot of food in small amounts often, might make it harder to stay energetic and aggravate arthritic symptoms.

Stabilizing Blood Sugar: It's important to keep regular eating habits, especially for people with reactive arthritis, to stabilize blood sugar levels. Frequent, evenly spaced meals and snacks throughout the day help avoid blood sugar spikes and falls, which can lower energy and perhaps exacerbate inflammation. Sophisticated carbs, when combined with lean proteins and good fats, help to maintain stable blood sugar levels.

Encouraging Nutrient Absorption: Eating regular, well-balanced meals promotes the best possible absorption of nutrients, guaranteeing that the body gets an adequate quantity of vital vitamins and minerals. This is especially crucial for people who have reactive arthritis because specific nutrients are essential Stabilizing Blood Sugar:

Encouraging Nutrient Absorption:

for reducing inflammation and maintaining joint health. Timing meals consistently promote the conditions necessary for the body to effectively absorb and use these nutrients.

Promoting Digestive Health: Eating regularly reduces the likelihood of gastrointestinal problems, which are frequently experienced by people with reactive arthritis. Consuming meals high in fiber, such as fruits, vegetables, and whole grains, helps maintain regular bowel movements and balanced gut flora. Additionally, proper hydration is necessary for healthy digestion and general well-being.

To sum up, creating nutrient-dense dishes, controlling portion sizes, and maintaining regular eating schedules are essential elements of the Reactive Arthritis Diet. Through the integration of diverse anti-inflammatory foods, individualization of quantities according to requirements, and adherence to regular eating routines, people can improve general health, alleviate symptoms, and improve their quality of life.

SECTION SIX

RECIPES FOR BRUNCH AND BREAKFAST

Boosting Smoothies for the Morning

Introduction: For people with reactive arthritis, it's critical to start your day with a nutrient-rich drink that contains anti-inflammatory components. Smoothies for an energetic start to the day are a delicious way to follow the guidelines of an arthritis-friendly diet.

Important Ingredients: When making these smoothies, pay attention to adding components that have anti-inflammatory qualities. Antioxidant-rich berries can be combined with leafy greens like spinach and kale. Add flaxseeds, ginger, and turmeric for an extra anti-inflammatory boost. The use of almond milk or coconut water as a base guarantees a dairy-free and arthritis-friendly base.

Recipes:

1. The Bliss Berry Smoothie:

• Combine a handful of spinach with a cup of mixed berries, including raspberries, strawberries, and blueberries.

• Include a tablespoon of flaxseed and a teaspoon of turmeric.

• For a revitalizing start to your day, use coconut water as the foundation.

2. Goddess Green Elixir:

• For a tropical twist, mix pineapple, cucumber, and greens.

• Add chia seeds and ginger for an added anti-inflammatory benefit.

• Almond milk provides a smooth, arthritic-friendly liquid foundation.

Customization Advice: Try different combinations to fit your dietary requirements and personal preferences. For more protein and creaminess, try adding a scoop of Greek yogurt or protein powder that is suitable for those with arthritis.

Breakfast Bowls and Parfaits Packed with Nutrition

Introduction: A visually pleasing and filling way to start your morning is with breakfast bowls and parfaits, which are a step up from smoothies. These nutrient-dense options meet the requirements of people on a reactive arthritis diet.

Grain-Free Granola Bowls: Make your grain-free granola instead of buying the packaged kind. To create a pleasant crunch without the inflammatory effects of grains, combine nuts, seeds, and dried fruits. Serve with a dollop of coconut yogurt and fresh berries for a tasty, arthritis-friendly breakfast.

Chia Seed Parfait: To make a chia seed parfait, add almonds and sliced fruits over chia pudding. Omega-3 fatty acids, which are abundant in chia seeds, have anti-inflammatory properties. Use dairy-free yogurt in between layers to improve flavor and texture while adhering to arthritis-friendly recommendations.

Sweet Potato Breakfast Bowl: The substantial foundation of a breakfast bowl is made of roasted sweet potatoes. For an added protein boost, top with avocado slices, sautéed vegetables, and a poached egg. This dish is nutrient-dense and a great option for people with reactive arthritis because of its fiber content, vitamins, and healthy fats.

Substitute Ingredients: If a person has dietary restrictions, take into account using substitute ingredients. Try making granola without gluten and replace conventional yogurt with yogurt made from coconut or almonds. Tailoring recipes to suit specific sensitivity levels guarantees a personalized and delightful morning meal.

Innovative and Tasty Brunch Selections

Introduction: If you're following a reactive arthritis diet, brunch is a great way to try new, delectable meals. These selections, which range from salty to sweet, prioritize joint health while satisfying a variety of palates.

Quinoa and Vegetable Frittata: Instead of using eggs, try making a frittata with quinoa, which is a high-protein substitute. Add as many vibrant veggies as you can, such as spinach, tomatoes, and bell peppers. Quinoa and vegetables work together to create a breakfast alternative that is both nutritious and arthritis-friendly. Varieties of Smashed Avocado Toast: Avocado toast is still a brunch staple and can be tailored to fit within an arthritis-friendly diet. Choose gluten-free bread and garnish it with cherry tomatoes, mashed avocado, and flaxseeds. This nutrient-dense choice is good for your joints and looks good too.

Tart with Salmon and Asparagus: Use omega-3 fatty acids by combining salmon with a flavorful tart. Add it to roasted asparagus and a gluten-free crust to make a wonderful brunch dish that helps support an anti-inflammatory diet.

Creative Drink Selections: Go ahead and serve your brunch fare with creative drinks like ginger-infused herbal teas or turmeric lattes. In addition to adding flair to your food, these drinks also have extra anti-inflammatory qualities, making your brunch experience more joint-friendly overall.

Conclusion: With these vibrant morning smoothies, nutrient-dense breakfast bowls, and delectable brunch alternatives, it's totally easy to strike a balance between creativity and following a reactive arthritis diet. Try out these recipes, and enjoy the satisfaction of cooking and eating meals that put joint health first without sacrificing flavor.

SECTION SEVEN

LUNCHES IN SUPPORT OF JOINT HEALTH

Bright Greens with reduced dressings

Salads as Allies for Joint Health

Bright salads can make a huge difference in your diet when it comes to joint health. Salads are a great source of critical vitamins and minerals that improve joint health and are packed with nutrients. When choosing leafy greens for your meal, go for a vibrant combination like spinach, kale, and arugula to add antioxidants that help fight inflammation. Add a range of veggies, such as tomatoes, cucumbers, and bell peppers, which have anti-inflammatory qualities and benefit joint health.

Anti-Inflammatory Dressings: Their Power

One of the most important parts of a reactive arthritis diet is to pair your colorful salads with anti-inflammatory dressings. Make dressings with components such as extra virgin olive oil, which has anti-inflammatory monounsaturated fats. Incorporate a small amount of turmeric, a strong anti-inflammatory spice, for added taste and health advantages. Take inspiration from the vivid colors of nature and add fresh herbs like parsley and cilantro to your dressings to boost the flavor and anti-inflammatory properties of your healthy meal.

Healthy Stems and Soups

Calm Soups for Combined Pain Relief

Rich soups are a top priority when it comes to joint health. Bone broth is a rich source of collagen and amino acids that maintain the health of joints and connective tissue. Use it as the foundation for hearty soups. Add veggies with anti-inflammatory qualities, such as celery, carrots, and sweet potatoes. For a meal that is well-rounded and nourishing for the joints, use lean proteins like fish or chicken. Soups, particularly those flavored with garlic and ginger, can provide an additional benefit by lowering inflammation and improving the health of all joints.

Stews: A Filling and Cooperative Choice

Not only are stews a soothing alternative, but they're also a great dietary choice for anyone looking to relieve joint pain. Choose plant-based proteins such as beans and lentils or lean meat cuts to up the protein content without sacrificing joint health. Steeping stews allow the flavors to mingle and the ingredients' nutritional value to be retained. To give your stew an extra anti-inflammatory boost and turn it into a tasty ally in the battle against reactive arthritis, try adding some turmeric and cayenne pepper.

Ideas for Handheld Lunches on Busy Days

Roll-ups and Wraps for Nutrition on the Go

Portable lunch options are essential for busy days. Roll-ups and wraps offer an easy and joint-friendly solution. Select wraps made of whole grains or gluten-free substitutes to accommodate particular dietary requirements. Stuff them full of colorful veggies and lean proteins like turkey or grilled chicken. Add avocado since it has monounsaturated fats that reduce inflammation and improve joint health in addition to making your lunch portable.

Quinoa and Vegetable Jars: A Powerful Treat Rich in Nutrients

Assemble nutrient-dense jars with layers of quinoa, roasted veggies, and leafy greens for a meal that is portable and supports joint health. As a complete protein, quinoa offers vital amino acids that promote general health. Vegetables that have been roasted enhance flavor and provide anti-inflammatory ingredients to the mixture. Put these jars together ahead of time for a quick and easy lunch choice that will help you stick to your reactive arthritis diet even on the busiest of days.

Personalized Trail Mix for Instant Energy

Make your joint-friendly trail mix for a simple and energizing lunch. Mix in nuts with anti-inflammatory qualities, such as walnuts and almonds, which are high in omega-3 fatty acids. Add some dried fruits, such as cherries, which have been shown to have anti-inflammatory properties. To add even more nutrients, add seeds like flaxseed and chia. For people with hectic schedules, this portable solution is ideal as it not only supports joint health but also offers consistent energy throughout the day.

In conclusion, a tasty and practical reactive arthritis diet can emphasize joint health. To make sure you keep a joint-friendly diet even on your busiest days, embrace the colorful world of salads and anti-inflammatory dressings, indulge in nutritious soups and stews, and choose portable lunch choices.

SECTION EIGHT

DINNERS THAT PROVIDE CALM

Filling One-Pot Dinners to Reduce Reactive Arthritis

A diet that not only promotes joint health but also makes eating enjoyable is necessary for those with reactive arthritis. One-pot meals become the perfect answer since they combine nutrition and ease of preparation. These recipes allow for a harmonious combination of foods that support an anti-inflammatory approach, while also minimizing the amount of preparation work required. With lean proteins like fish or chicken and a rainbow of bright veggies, one-pot wonders make a filling and simple-to-digest dinner choice.

Quinoa stew with chicken and vegetables

Start your cooking adventure with a filling bowl of chicken and vegetable quinoa stew. The foundation is made of quinoa, a grain devoid of gluten and high in vital nutrients that serve as a healthy substitute for grains. Add lean chicken, which is high in anti-inflammatory properties, and a variety of vibrant veggies, such as carrots, bell peppers, and spinach. This stew is an excellent one-pot meal for those with reactive arthritis because it not only tastes great but also benefits joint health.

Sweet Potato Casserole with Salmon

Try a salmon and sweet potato casserole for a boost of omega-3 fatty acids and anti-inflammatory properties. Sweet potatoes offer complex carbohydrates and flavor, while salmon's high omega-3 concentration reduces inflammation. This combination of ingredients is guaranteed by the one-pot casserole method, which results in a dish that not only calms the palate but also meets the unique nutritional requirements of those with reactive arthritis.

Plant-Based and Vegetarian Dinner Ideas for Joint Health

Changing supper to a vegetarian or plant-based meal not only accommodates people with dietary restrictions but also has many advantages for people with reactive arthritis. These foods, which are rich in fiber, antioxidants, and other vital nutrients, support a diet low in inflammation and improve joint health and general well-being.

Lentil and Mushroom Stuffed Peppers

With these stuffed peppers made with mushrooms and lentils, discover the world of plant-based nourishment. Lentils are a protein-rich legume that goes well with mushrooms, which are well-known for strengthening the immune system. Together, they make a tasty and filling stuffing. Bell peppers are an excellent source of vitamins and antioxidants. This dish is a great option for people who are looking for relief from reactive arthritis because it not only satisfies the palate but also displays the range and inventiveness of vegetarian cuisine.

Curry with Chickpeas and Spinach

Savor the flavor of a chickpea and spinach curry, which is aromatic and spicy. Protein-rich chickpeas and nutrient-dense spinach combine in a delicious spice blend. This vegan curry guarantees a bountiful supply of vital nutrients while also satisfying the craving for strong flavors. It's a smart choice for people who want to manage reactive arthritis while having a filling and substantial dinner because of the anti-inflammatory qualities of the components.

Succulent Grilled and Roasted Treats for Cozy Dinners

Meals are given a unique flavor profile by grilling and roasting methods, which also maintain the nutritional value of the foods. For those coping with the difficulties of reactive arthritis, grilling, and roasting foods guarantees a tasty meal without sacrificing joint health.

Spiced Grilled Chicken with Herbs

Herb-infused grilled Chicken is a scrumptious dish that blends the ease of grilling with the aromatic appeal of fresh herbs to elevate your dinner. This recipe is great for joints since it has high-quality protein from chicken and anti-inflammatory herbs like thyme and rosemary. For reactive arthritis sufferers, grilling adds a smokey taste while maintaining nutritional content, making for a delicious and health-conscious supper.

Spiced Roasted Vegetable Medley

In a Roasted Vegetable Medley, harness the power of colorful veggies and the anti-inflammatory spice turmeric. This recipe combines a vibrant mix of perfectly roasted veggies, including bell peppers, zucchini, and carrots. Turmeric is added, which not only adds a warming, earthy flavor but also helps control inflammation. This roast beauty is a great option for anyone looking for reactive arthritis diet meal ideas because it is not only aesthetically pleasing but also a nutritional powerhouse.

SECTION NINE

SNACKS FOR COLLABORATION

Ideas for Nutrient-Dense Snacks to Support Each Other

The significance of nutrient-dense snacks for diet-based management of reactive arthritis cannot be emphasized. These snacks are crucial for supplying important vitamins and minerals that support healthy joints. Choosing nutrient-dense foods guarantees that your body gets the nutrition it needs without adding extraneous ingredients that could worsen inflammation.

A handful of mixed nuts makes a great snack that is high in nutrients. Nuts like walnuts and almonds, which are rich in antioxidants and omega-3 fatty acids, help to lessen joint inflammation. They also supply a sufficient amount of calcium and magnesium, which strengthens bones.

A healthy snack idea is a Greek yogurt topped with fresh berries. Probiotics and protein found in Greek yogurt help maintain digestive health, which is related to joint health. Berries, which are high in antioxidants, contribute to the snack's anti-inflammatory qualities, making it a tasty and nutritious option for people with reactive arthritis.

Handmade Energy Bites and Trail Mixes

Making your own energy bites or trail mix lets you customize the ingredients to fit the requirements of a reactive arthritis diet. These homemade snacks provide the ideal ratio of fiber, protein, and good fats, which supports healthy joints and maintains energy levels throughout the day.

Trail Mix for Arthritis:

Consider mixing dried fruits, seeds, and unsalted nuts in a homemade trail mix. Nuts supply vital omega-3 fatty acids, seeds such as flaxseed and chia offer fiber and anti-inflammatory qualities, and dried fruits contribute extra nutrients and a naturally pleasant taste. Since maintaining a healthy weight is essential for joint health, take care when determining portion sizes to prevent consuming too many calories.

Recipe for Energy Bites:

Making your energy bites at home is a fun and fulfilling way to have a healthy snack. A basic dish could use chia seeds, honey, almond butter, and rolled oats. You may add extra personalization to these bites by adding things like dark chocolate chips or dried fruits. As a good source of soluble fiber, oats may help reduce inflammation and support digestive health.

Including Fresh Vegetables and Fruits

A reactive arthritis diet should include a lot of fresh fruits and vegetables because they are rich in vitamins, minerals, and antioxidants. By adding them to snacks, you can improve their nutritional content while also supporting general joint health.

Hummus on vibrant vegetable sticks:

Cut a variety of vibrant veggies, such as cucumbers, carrots, and bell peppers, into sticks and serve with homemade hummus. The vivid colors represent many antioxidants, each of which has a specific function in lowering inflammation. Chickpea-based hummus promotes joint health by offering protein and important minerals like zinc and iron.

Fruit Skewers with a Sweet Finish:

Make fruit kabobs using a selection of berries, pineapple chunks, and melon slices for a naturally sweet snack. A class of antioxidants with anti-inflammatory qualities called anthocyanins is found in berries, especially strawberries and blueberries. The assortment of fruits adds various vitamins and enzymes that support the general health of joints.

In summary, the inclusion of fresh fruits and vegetables, nutrient-dense snacks, and handmade trail mixes should be the top priorities of a reactive arthritis diet that emphasizes joint care. As part of their overall dietary approach, people can actively help manage inflammation and promote joint health by carefully choosing and preparing these snacks.

SECTION TEN

SWEETS WITH A WELLNESS ORIENTATION

Sugary Goodies without the Resentment

Reactive arthritis sufferers must be aware of their nutrition, even when it comes to enjoying sweets. Luckily, the "Reactive Arthritis Diet Cook Book" offers a range of guilt-free dessert choices that fulfill your sweet taste while also adhering to the nutritional recommendations for reactive arthritis management.

Finding Sugar Substitutes: Using sugar substitutes wisely is a crucial part of creating desserts with a health-conscious twist. Those who have reactive arthritis should be concerned as traditional refined sugar might exacerbate inflammation. The cookbook offers a delicious balance between sweetness and health by examining natural sweeteners like honey, maple syrup, and agave nectar. These substitutions not only improve taste but also supply necessary nutrients, so your dessert won't interfere with your diet.

Including healthy Grains: Including healthy grains is another way the cookbook reimagines desserts. Among the many health advantages of whole grains are their anti-inflammatory qualities. Desserts made with oats or whole grain flour have a lovely texture and improve joint health overall. These selections demonstrate how a reactive arthritis-friendly diet can be both delicious and health-conscious, ranging from whole wheat cakes to oat-based cookies.

Accepting Nutrient-Rich Ingredients: When making desserts, the cookbook promotes using nutrient-rich ingredients. Nuts, seeds, and dark chocolate are among the ingredients that enhance the flavor profile and supply vital vitamins and minerals that promote joint health. You are fueling your body as well as your taste senses when you incorporate these ingredients into your sweet treats. Desserts Made with Fruit and Frozen Treats

In the "Reactive Arthritis Diet Cook Book," fruits take center stage in delectable and nourishing dessert recipes, making them the heroes of the story. Through the use of fruits' inherent sweetness and anti-inflammatory qualities, these recipes present a wonderful substitute for customary sweets.

The Bright World of Fruit Salads: This cookbook offers a completely fresh perspective on fruit salads. These salads, which combine a range of fruits high in vitamins and antioxidants, are not only bursting with flavor but also help lower inflammation. There are countless options for sweet and tart citrus fruits as well as sweet berries, making them a vibrant and nutrient-rich dessert choice.

Chilled Delights for Joint Comfort: This cookbook delves into the world of icy delicacies, with a focus on frozen desserts. Sorbets and fruit-based popsicles are examples of chilled treats that soothe sore joints in addition to cooling your palette. Desserts made with fruits that have anti-inflammatory qualities are a great option for those with reactive arthritis since they provide a cool, soothing treat.

Smoothies as Nutrient-Rich Desserts: Several nutrient-dense smoothies that can be served as desserts are presented in the cookbook. Smoothies that combine anti-inflammatory fruits with healthy ingredients like chia seeds and yogurt provide a guilt-free yet wholesome way to enjoy sweets. They offer a tasty way to have a satisfying dessert and include nutrients that are good for your joints in your diet.

Luxurious yet Anti-Inflammatory Choices

Unlike what many people think, indulgence is acceptable in a reactive arthritis-friendly diet. The "Reactive Arthritis Diet Cook Book" offers a variety of decadent, anti-inflammatory dessert choices that address joint health concerns as well as comfort.

Decadent Dark Chocolate Delights: The cookbook features dark chocolate as the main ingredient and a guilt-free treat. Desserts made with dark chocolate, which is high in antioxidants and has anti-inflammatory qualities, are now considered opulent but health-conscious options. These alternatives, which range from velvety mousse to rich truffles, demonstrate that enjoyment may be combined with a reactive arthritis diet.

Creative Use of Spices: Known for their anti-inflammatory qualities, the cookbook offers a variety of spices. Ginger, turmeric, and cinnamon become essential ingredients in dessert recipes, enhancing flavor and benefiting joint health. Rich pastries flavored with these spices are a creative way to manage reactive arthritis through nutrition in addition to being a tantalizing treat for the palate.

Low-Glycemic Sweeteners for Dessert Bliss: No need to worry about blood sugar spikes after indulging in sweets. The cookbook looks at ways to enjoy sweets without sacrificing health by using low-glycemic sweeteners like stevia and monk fruit. For those who are managing reactive arthritis, these sweeteners provide a safe substitute that lets them enjoy desserts without worrying about aggravating inflammation.

To sum up, the "Reactive Arthritis Diet Cook Book" goes above and beyond limitations, proving that desserts can promote joint health and be a source of enjoyment. This cookbook redefines the sweet side of a reactive arthritis-friendly diet by embracing anti-inflammatory alternatives, emphasizing fruits, and combining inventive ingredients that make every indulgence a delightful and thoughtful experience.

SECTION ELEVEN

DRINKS TO PROMOTE JOINT HEALTH

The Effects of Hydration on Joint Health

Introduction: Maintaining adequate hydration is essential to leading a health-conscious lifestyle. It is particularly important for people with reactive arthritis as it plays a major role in joint health management. Maintaining joint lubrication, reducing the force on cartilage, and promoting the delivery of nutrients to the impacted areas all depend on drinking enough water.

Water: The Elixir of Joint Wellness: Essential to maintaining healthy joints, water serves as more than just a means of slaking thirst. Maintaining an ideal daily water consumption is essential for a reactive arthritis diet. Water aids in the removal of toxins from the body, lowering inflammation and enhancing joint comfort in general. Sufficient hydration is also necessary for synovial fluid, which lubricates joints and lowers friction, to function properly.

Including Hydrating Foods: Adding hydrating foods to your diet is a smart way to promote joint health in addition to drinking plenty of water. Foods like cucumber, celery, and watermelon that are high in water content can help you meet your daily fluid needs. Including these in your diet helps to relieve joint soreness by providing important nutrients and hydrating the body.

Electrolyte Balancing for Joint Support: Electrolytes are essential for preserving the body's fluid equilibrium. Calcium, magnesium, potassium, sodium, and other vital electrolytes support healthy joints. To maximize hydration in a reactive arthritis diet, it's critical to balance these electrolytes. Foods high in potassium, such as spinach and bananas, can be especially helpful in preserving joint health.

Limiting Dehydrating Beverages: Some drinks might worsen joint pain by dehydrating the body. Drinking sugary and caffeinated beverages in moderation is recommended for those with reactive arthritis. These drinks may increase fluid loss and perhaps exacerbate joint pain due to their diuretic properties. Choosing water infused with fruits and herbs and herbal teas becomes a more beneficial option for joint health.

Teas & Infusions for Healing

The Healing Potential of Herbal Teas: Traditionally prized for their therapeutic qualities, herbal teas can provide a calming effect on swollen joints when included in a reactive arthritis diet. Due to its anti-inflammatory qualities, ginger tea can help reduce joint discomfort. Another effective choice that has been shown to have the ability to relieve pain and reduce inflammation is turmeric tea, which is high in curcumin.

Infusions of Mint and Chamomile: Infusions of Mint and Chamomile not only have a delicious flavor, but they also have a relaxing effect on joints. Because of its anti-inflammatory and antioxidant qualities, chamomile tea is a helpful ally in the treatment of reactive arthritis symptoms. Mint is a delightful option for people looking for a natural approach to joint wellness because of its cooling feeling, which can help relieve inflammatory joints.

Green Tea for an Antioxidant Boost: Rich in antioxidants such as catechins, green tea can be a useful supplement to a diet for reactive arthritis. By lowering oxidative stress in the body, these antioxidants may be able to lessen joint inflammation. Everyday routines that include a cup of green tea can help provide the general antioxidant support that is essential for joint health.

Nettle Tea: Nature's Anti-Inflammatory Herbal Remedies: Made from the stinging nettle plant, nettle tea is a little-known but effective treatment for inflammation of the joints. It has ingredients that have anti-inflammatory qualities that could lessen the symptoms of arthritis. Including nettle tea in your drink routine offers a comprehensive and all-natural way to promote joint health.

Smoothies to Refresh and Support Joints

Overview of Joint-Friendly Smoothies: Smoothies are a great way to get nutrients that support joint health in addition to being a tasty treat. Reactive arthritis diets can benefit from the tasty and nourishing inclusion of smoothies made with components recognized for their anti-inflammatory and joint-supportive qualities.

Berry Blast Antioxidant Smoothie: Antioxidants, which are abundant in berries like raspberries, strawberries, and blueberries, help fight oxidative stress. Smoothies high in antioxidants may help to lessen joint inflammation. These berries make a cool, satisfying drink that is suitable for sharing as a snack or for breakfast when combined with a base of almond milk or coconut water.

Combination of Pineapple and Turmeric: Pineapple, with its enzyme bromelain, and turmeric, with its anti-inflammatory ingredient curcumin, work well together to relieve joint pain. Combining pieces of pineapple, coconut milk, a pinch of honey, and a sprinkle of turmeric into a blender creates a tropical smoothie that is not only delicious but also helps to reduce joint inflammation.

Avocado and Leafy Greens Elixir: When avocado and leafy greens like spinach and kale are combined, a nutrient-rich smoothie is produced. These greens are a great source of vitamins and minerals that help maintain healthy joints. The avocado contributes to joint lubrication by adding a serving of good fats. A tasty method to include these nutrients in your diet that are good for your joints is to blend them into a smoothie.

Protein-Packed Almond Butter Banana Smoothie: Healthy muscles and joints depend on consuming enough protein. When combined with banana, and almond butter—high in protein and good fats—makes for a delicious combo that promotes healthy joint function. The smoothie's nutritional profile is improved by adding a scoop of protein powder, which makes it a gratifying and nutritious choice for people with reactive arthritis.

In summary, creating a reactive arthritis diet that prioritizes healing teas, cool smoothies, and plenty of water can make a big difference in joint health. Including these drinks in your daily routine gives you vital nutrients and gives your pursuit of ideal joint health a tasty and pleasurable twist.

SECTION TWELVE

GOING BEYOND THE RECIPE BOOK

Including Long-Term Lifestyle Adjustments

Since reactive arthritis is a chronic ailment, symptom management and general well-being enhancement necessitate a comprehensive strategy. Achieving long-lasting relief and encouraging a healthier lifestyle needs embracing long-term lifestyle adjustments.

Balanced Nutrition: Eating a diet high in anti-inflammatory foods is essential for treating reactive arthritis. Give lean proteins, omega-3 fatty acids, and a rainbow of colorful fruits and vegetables a priority. Legumes and whole grains can minimize triggers that could worsen symptoms while still offering vital nutrients. To create a diet plan that is customized to your unique requirements, think about speaking with a nutritionist.

Hydration Matters: Sufficient hydration is essential for maintaining joint health and normal physiological processes. Water facilitates digestion, removes toxins from the body, and keeps joints lubricated. Make a conscious effort to drink plenty of water throughout the day rather than sugar-filled drinks. Herbal teas can reduce inflammation and improve hydration levels.

Regular Exercise: Maintaining muscle strength and joint flexibility requires incorporating an appropriate exercise program into your everyday routine. Exercises with less impact, including yoga, walking, and swimming, can be especially helpful. Speak with a fitness expert or physiotherapist to create a customized workout program that fits your unique needs and builds up to a progressive intensity.

Making Sleep a Priority: The body's regeneration and repair processes depend on getting enough good sleep. Make sure your surroundings are sleep-friendly and stick to a regular sleep routine. To promote joint comfort, spend money on pillows and a comfy mattress. If your sleep problems don't go away, think about seeing a doctor to treat any possible underlying problems.

Stress Management Techniques: Stress can make chronic illnesses worse, such as reactive arthritis. Include stress-relieving activities in your everyday routine, such as mindfulness, deep breathing techniques, or meditation. Reading, gardening, or spending time with loved ones are examples of enjoyable hobbies that can have a favorable effect on your mental and physical health.

Keeping Yourself Inspired During Your Reactive Arthritis Path

Maintaining motivation is crucial for sticking to lifestyle modifications and attaining long-term success when dealing with reactive arthritis. Your capacity to properly handle symptoms can be greatly impacted by acknowledging the difficulties and putting solutions in place to maintain motivation.

Setting Achievable Short- and Long-Term Goals: Set attainable goals that complement your overall health objectives. Appreciate the little things that go well along the way, like more flexibility in your joints or effectively following a diet. A sense of accomplishment from reaching realistic goals encourages perseverance in the pursuit of improved health.

Creating a Support System: Be in the company of friends, family, and medical professionals who are sympathetic to your situation. Tell them about your objectives, and rely on them when things go tough. Having a network of support can help you stay motivated to manage your reactive arthritis by offering you emotional, practical, and encouraging support.

Monitoring Your Progress: Keep a notebook to record your symptoms, food selections, workout regimens, and general state of health. Examining your development regularly can assist in identifying trends, triggers, and opportunities for development. In addition to providing you with new perspectives, this reflective exercise acts as a tangible reminder of your progress.

Educating Yourself: Keep up with the most recent findings in research as well as information regarding reactive arthritis and available treatments. Knowing gives you strength and enables you to make wise decisions regarding your well-being. Join support groups, webinars, or seminars to meet people going through similar things and learn insightful things.

Extra Sources and Additional Reading

Increasing your knowledge and getting access to more resources are essential if you want to effectively manage reactive arthritis. You may improve your general well-being and make educated decisions about your health with the help of an informed approach.

Medical providers and Specialists: It's critical to build trusting relationships with rheumatologists, dietitians, and physical therapists, among other healthcare providers. Frequent examinations, honest dialogue, and teamwork with experts can all help create a thorough and individualized treatment plan that caters to your unique requirements.

Support Groups and Communities: Participating in online communities or support groups for reactive arthritis offers a priceless chance to meet people going through comparable struggles. Emotional support and useful insights can be obtained by exchanging experiences, advice, and coping mechanisms. These groups frequently provide inspiration and understanding.

Trustworthy Publications and Websites: Look through credible publications, websites, and research articles about reactive arthritis and related subjects. Keep up on the most recent developments in medicine, available treatments, and suggested lifestyles. When it comes to taking care of your health and making wise decisions, knowledge is a valuable asset.

Books and Educational Resources: Read books and educational resources authored by professionals in the area to deepen your awareness of reactive arthritis. These sites can offer a comprehensive understanding of the ailment, its underlying causes, and practical management techniques. Seek out publications that are supported by respectable medical associations and adhere to evidence-based methods.

In summary, managing the intricacies of reactive arthritis necessitates accepting long-term lifestyle adjustments, maintaining your motivation throughout the process, and persistently looking for new resources to broaden your understanding. Combining these components will provide you the ability to effectively control your symptoms and live a full life despite the difficulties that reactive arthritis presents.

Made in the USA
Coppell, TX
24 June 2024